Honey Diet

40+ Benefits and Uses of Honey

Rachel Gemba

Table of Contents

Introduction 3

Chapter 1: The Lowdown on Honey 4

Chapter 2: The 40 + Benefits and Uses of Honey 6

Conclusion 16

Your Free Gift

I am really grateful and thankful for your purchase. As a small symbol of my appreciation, I would like to give you my FREE book on Essential Oils so you can begin to use them in your life.

In my essential oils: 100+ Essential Oils for beauty, healing, personal care, and detox ebook, you will find various ways and methods that will help you to use essential oils and get results RIGHT NOW. You will also get all my new ebooks at a discounted price ☺

Here is the link for the ebook:

Download Now

Introduction

Do you have a sweet tooth? If you do, then you will find that a diet laced with honey is just the thing to get you into the prime of health while at the same time satiating your cravings for sweet sensations.

One doesn't necessarily have to have a sweet tooth where it comes to adopting that honey diet as a part of one's lifestyle, though. All one has to see is the vast plethora of benefits that a honey diet can afford you, so that one can rest assured that they are taking exactly the right decision where it comes to optimizing their health with something that is one hundred percent natural and has a wide range of benefits and uses that will all work superbly to our advantage.

Are you ready to find out just how good that honey diet can be for you where it comes to taking your health to the next level? Let's dive straight into the contents of this book, then, and extract the vital information we need, just like the precious honey that is the talk of this book, is retrieved from that beehive!

Chapter 1: The Lowdown on Honey

You will find that a tablespoon of raw honey is completely free of fat, cholesterol and sodium and contains only 64 calories, according to the National Honey Board. It has been used way back in the time of the Egyptian tombs, on account of its widely touted antibacterial and antifungal properties. This golden fluid is indeed gold where it comes to providing the human body with a whole host of benefits that can improve the quality of our health by a great extent.

It's not only humans out there who have been raiding those beehives out there for years. A lot of animals, including bears and badgers, have been constantly attacking beehives in order to delight in the wonderful sweet spoils that are contained within them.

Honey was actually the most widely used natural sweetener until the sixteenth century, when sugar was made available for consumption to the general public.

How honey is made

Before we start let's get into the wonderful benefits that honey affords us, let's take a quick look at exactly how honey is made in the very first place!

It starts with nectar

Honey starts as nectar from flowers – this nectar is collected by bees and stored in their honeycombs after it has been broken down into simple sugars. The bees fan their wings and enable the process of evaporation to happen, thus resulting in the golden viscous fluid that we know to be honey.

Then come the beekeepers

It's a good thing that bees produce far more honey than is required by them. Thus, the excess is available for our use without us having to feel guilty about it. It's the beekeeper who comes in next – they collect the honeycomb frames and scrape off the wax caps that seal the honey in each cell. The frames are then placed in an extractor that helps to squeeze the honey out of the comb.

The final process

In the end it's time to strain the honey to remove any pieces of wax that might still be there. After that it is time to bottle the honey and send it to the retailers who will sell them to people out there. You might wish to purchase a bottle of pure honey, so that you can be assured that what you are getting is nothing short of being one hundred percent unadulterated honey.

Chapter 2: The 40 + Benefits and Uses of Honey

Now that we've gotten a little lowdown on honey and discovered exactly how it is made, it's time to take a look at all the wonderful benefits and uses of the wonderful golden liquid, so that we can know exactly how effective that honey diet of ours can really be!

The 40 + Benefits and Uses of Honey

#1 It is good for your blood. You will find that when you mix honey in tepid water, it has this amazing effect of increasing the red blood cell count in the body. This helps people who have anemic conditions, by increasing the oxygen-carrying capability of the blood. People who have decreased oxygen-carrying capability in their blood often suffer from fatigue and breathlessness and a honey-based diet helps offset these conditions. It also helps to relieve hypertension, which is a most serious problem these days.

#2 It's useful as a pore cleanser. You will find that the enzymes in raw honey help to keep your pores clean. Besides, the antibacterial properties of honey ensure that there are no breakouts on your skin. All you have to do is add one tablespoon of honey to two tablespoons of coconut oil, and massage the mixture onto your face while avoiding the eyes. Then make sure that you rinse the application off with tepid water.

#3 It helps to combat hangovers. You will find that if you wake up groggy in the morning with a hangover, you can combat its effects by mixing a little bit of honey (around 15ml) in around 80 ml of orange juice. Add 70 ml of natural yogurt to these two and blend them all together until you get a rather smooth mixture. Drink this and you will see that the fructose(natural sugar) in honey will help speed up the oxidation of alcohol by the liver, thus helping you sober up well before time.

#4 It gives you a lot of essential nutrients. Quite simply one of the simplest reasons to have more honey in your diet is because of the vast array of nutrients it provides you with. You will find that you get a lot of vitamins and minerals like zinc, riboflavin, copper, magnesium and iron, thus ensuring that you get far more value where it comes to using honey as a sweetening agent, as opposed to using sugar, which only provides you with empty calories.

#5 It's a great energy drink. If you are looking to get a quick boost of energy that is not going to increase that caloric count of yours, then you want to use honey – you will find that the fructose and glucose in it quickly enter your bloodstream and give you exactly the boost you needed, while at the very same time ensuring that you are not ingesting more than 17 grams of carbohydrates per tablespoon.

#6 It's great in the treatment of wounds. Honey is antibacterial and antiseptic, and hence can be extremely effective where it comes to the treatment of wounds. In fact, it is one of the oldest known wound dressings in the world. You will find that inflammation, swelling and even pain dramatically subside after honey has been applied to the wounded area. Because it is anti-inflammatory it is also an excellent choice where it comes to the treatment of burns.

#7 It's good to use as a moisturizing mask. You don't need to go to the spa to avail of that moisturizing mask. Honey is an excellent choice where it comes to creating the very same, because it draws moisture from the air that can be retained in the skin to provide hydration that is long lasting. You will see that you can easily create a natural moisturizing mask by spreading one teaspoon of honey on dry, clean skin and letting it sit there for a period of 15 minutes before washing it off with tepid water.

#8 It helps in the improvement of diabetes. You will find that not only can honey help in assisting medication in the case of those people who are living with diabetes, but it can also help in the prevention of the same. This is because raw honey increases insulin in the body and reduces hyperglycemia. All you have to do is add raw honey to your diet and observe the reaction of your your blood sugar to it over time!

#9 It helps in fighting off cold. Using buckwheat-based honey syrup can be just the thing you needed, where it comes to keeping that cold of yours at bay. Research has shown that using a syrup of this kind was more effective in easing the nighttime cough of children and helping to aid in their sleeping, in comparison to the normal cough syrup you get over the counter at the chemist. The honey syrup is really marvelous in helping to fight off infection.

#10 It can help to improve your scalp. Seborrheic dermatitis is a condition that is responsible for causing dandruff and itching in your scalp. All you have to do is dilute honey with a little bit of warm water and apply the solution to your scalp once every other day for the period of four weeks. You will find that not only will the itching be relieved in a short time, but there will also be a significant improvement in hair loss, if there is any.

#11 It can be used for your eyes. The ancient Egyptians and Indians used honey most effectively in the treatment of eye diseases. You will find that you can treat eye conditions like redness and itching of the eyes and conjunctivitis, among others, using honey. In fact, it is also touted as being a good means for the prevention of cataract. All you have to do is dissolve honey in warm water. When the solution cools, apply it as an eye bath!

#12 It helps to build your immune system. You will find that honey is rather excellent where it comes to help build that immune system of yours, on account of its anti-oxidant properties. All you need to do is squeeze the juice of half a lemon with a teaspoon of honey first thing in the morning, and drink it. Make sure you establish this as a regular practice and you will be boosting that immune system of yours by a great extent.

#13 It helps kill bacteria that are resistant to antibiotics. People get rather desperate when the antibiotics they are using to kill the bacteria in their system do not work, and honey could just be the perfect solution for their needs. You will find that medical grade honey can really work wonders where it comes to killing dangerous pathogens like E. Coli and salmonella that are otherwise very resistant to antibiotics. This has been verified by clinical studies.

#14 It helps in overall brain function. The antioxidants that honey is rich in help to prevent cellular loss and damage in the brain. If you consume honey regularly, you will surely have better short-term memory than if you don't. Honey also has the ability to help the body absorb calcium, and this is really good where it comes to helping us process thought and make decisions, as calcium is needed by the brain for those very reasons. This can also help in the long run to stave off dementia.

#15 It helps in the process of digestion. Honey is a mild laxative and is therefore great where it comes to aiding the process of digestion. You will find that things like constipation, gas and bloating can be most effectively treated, through the simple consumption of honey. It is also helpful in the promotion of digestion because it is rich in probiotic bacteria like lactobacilli. When you use honey in place of table sugar, you will find that you reduce the risk of toxic effect in the gut that are caused by fungi.

#16 It helps reduce scars on the face. Honey is known to reduce facial scars on account of its skin-lightening properties. The anti-inflammatory and antibacterial properties it has help in tissue regeneration and healing. Mix a teaspoon of raw honey with a teaspoon of coconut oil and apply it in a circular motion to the affected area for one or two minutes. Then apply a hot washcloth to it and let it sit until it cools. Do this daily until you get the desired results!

#17 It helps you sleep better. For all those people out there who are having a rather difficult time coping with insomnia, you will find that honey is exactly what the doctor ordered. The thing is, honey helps the body release serotonin, which is a neurotransmitter that helps improve your mood. Furthermore, the serotonin this released is converted into melatonin, which is a chemical compound that is integral where it comes to regulating the quality and the length of one's sleep!

#18 It's excellent in the treatment of herpes. This is because the high sugar content in honey helps prevent the growth of microorganisms in your wound. Moreover, honey also draws fluid from the same and also releases low levels of hydrogen peroxide when the honey comes into contact with your wound. The commonly prescribed antiviral cream for Herpes is Acyclovir, and one study found that the application of honey was far more effective where it came to the treatment of both labial and genital herpes.

#19 It helps in weight loss. You would never quite imagine that something sweet could ever be able to assist you in the process of weight loss, right? Well, a honey-based diet is just the thing you need to shed those extra pounds. The thing is this – in order to digest sugar, a lot of vitamins and minerals that would otherwise be most helpful in dissolving fats, are utilized. Hence, when one replaces that sugar with honey they will find that they keep those critical vitamins and minerals, very much intact to burn those fats in your body.

#20 It helps in the treatment of dandruff. Tired of that dandruff in your hair? Apply some honey diluted with ten percent warm water to your hair and rinse it after three hours. Its antibacterial and antifungal properties will ensure it takes care of that dandruff that is caused by an overgrowth of fungus.

#21 It helps prevent and control cancer. What most people are not aware about, is that honey has carcinogenic-preventing and anti-tumor properties, which make it an excellent choice in the treatment and prevention of cancer. So, whether you have cancer or not, infusing your diet with more honey indeed makes a lot of sense where it comes to fighting the world's deadliest disease.

#22 It helps to reduce ulcers and gastrointestinal disorders. Thanks to the antibacterial properties of honey, it is really an excellent choice where it comes to the treatment of ulcers and other gastrointestinal disorders. This is largely on account of the hydrogen peroxide that is released from the honey as we have touched upon earlier. In fact, it is interesting to note that the bees add an enzyme to the honey that is responsible for the release of the said hydrogen peroxide.

#23 It helps to improve athletic performance. We have already seen that honey can give one a quick boost of energy, but what's really interesting is the fact that it can be very beneficial to athletes because it helps muscles recover after that workout and also helps to restore glycogen levels that have been depleted. It also regulates the expenditure of energy in the body, thereby making it an excellent choice for those with an athletic streak.

#24 It may help to relieve seasonal allergies. Although this hasn't been proven by clinical studies, it has been observed that honey could be just the thing you needed to combat those allergies, thanks to the traces of flower pollen it contains.

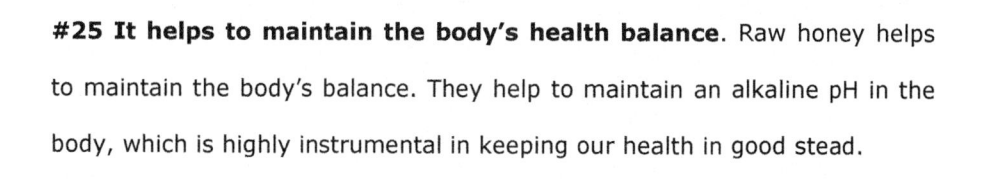

#25 It helps to maintain the body's health balance. Raw honey helps to maintain the body's balance. They help to maintain an alkaline pH in the body, which is highly instrumental in keeping our health in good stead.

#26 It can be used as an antibacterial soap. There are several skin infections that you could easily stave off, simply by using that honey as an antibacterial soap instead of the regular bar of soap you use in your home.

#27 It helps to speed up the growth of that healthy tissue. Honey can be great in ensuring your tissues are kept healthy thanks to the amino acids and vitamin C that are found in it.

#28 It's great for invigorating starts in the morning. Thanks to the abundant source of liver glycogen that honey provides you, it's a great way to start that morning of yours with an invigorating burst of energy!

#29 It helps to regulate the level of cholesterol in the body. Have a high level of that bad cholesterol? Incorporating more honey in your diet might be just the thing you need, as it is very effective in regulating the cholesterol level in the body.

#30 It helps in the treatment of acne. Tired of getting acne all the time and finding that there is little you can do about it? Well, try honey! Simply apply it to the affected area and let it sit for fifteen minutes or so, before washing it off with tepid water.

#31 It helps in the healing of sunburn. You don't carry sunscreen everywhere and in the times that you cannot escape that sunburn out there, you could do very well by applying honey to the affected area and leaving it for some time. Watch how well your skin will heal in the process!

#32 It helps in the prevention of ageing. Want to look younger for longer? Well, honey is just the thing you needed. The antioxidants it contains helps to protect that body of yours from the cell damage that is caused by free radicals, which are responsible for the very process of ageing itself. So, if you're not getting enough fruits and vegetables into your diet (to get the very same antioxidants), don't stress. All you need is to up your intake of honey and you will find yourself getting the very same results in the process!

#33 It helps to maintain the health of your heart. Your heart's health is something that needs to be taken very seriously, and you can do just that by ensuring that you have a high honey intake that will enable you to keep your heart in good health thanks to the homocysteine-level-reducing properties of honey.

#34 It helps in relieving the symptoms of stomach upset and nausea. If you have eaten something outside that has not agreed well with you, make sure you reach out for that dollop of honey in order to ensure that you bring that discomfort caused by stomach upset and nausea to a minimum.

#35 Use it as a hair conditioner. You can use honey as a very effective means of conditioning your hair, when you combine it with coconut oil. You will find that the enzymes and the nutrients in honey will help give that much needed shine to that dull hair of yours, while that coconut oil will help to smoothen the hair cuticles. Now mix one spoon of honey(raw) with 2 spoons of coconut oil, and then apply it to damp hair. Let it sit for 20 minutes prior to washing it off.

#36 It helps to fight indigestion. If you find that you are suffering from indigestion, then a very simple solution would be to take a couple of teaspoons of honey, that will help make sure that your digestive process is most effectively bolstered as a result.

#37 It helps in the soothing of a sore throat. We have already seen the wonders that honey can work for colds, but it also has a great effect in the case of coughs. You will find that if you add a teaspoon or two to hot tea with lemon, it can work wonderfully in the process of soothing that sore throat of yours. What's more, it has been proven to be as effective a cough suppressant as dextromethorphan, which is an over- the –counter cough medication.

#38 It improves blood circulation. Besides maintaining a healthy heart, honey also helps to regulate blood circulation, which is essential for our overall health and functioning.

#39 It helps in combating acid reflux. If you have an acid reflux problem, then you will find that honey can be a very good weapon for you where it comes to combating the same.

#40 It can be used as a natural sweetener, but make sure you get it from a reliable source. The best part about using honey is, of course, the fact that it can be used as a natural sweetener. Make sure that all the sugar in your diet is replaced by honey, but when you do make sure that you get it from a trusted source like *Trader Joe's*, in order to ensure that what you are getting is only one hundred percent raw honey.

#41 It can be combined with your shampoo for the best possible results. When it comes to using a shampoo, you want a really good one – one that will not only clean your hair well, but that will moisturize it well enough as well as strengthen it. Thanks to the humectant properties of honey, you will find that your hair is well moisturized. Besides, honey will also help in the process of strengthening your hair. All you need to do is mix a little bit of shampoo with a teaspoon of honey and then wash and rinse your hair like you normally would. Then all you need to do is sit back and watch the results unfold beautifully over time.

#42 It helps in keeping that constipation at bay. If you suffer from constipation then you will find that you can very well relieve that constipation of yours by mixing some apple cider vinegar with honey and consuming it. This will ensure that your constipation problem is well taken care of!

#43 It can be used to prevent headaches. If you suffer from recurrent headaches, you will find that if you use the brand of eucalyptus honey, then you will be ensuring that you prevent those headaches of yours from coming on every now and then.

#44 It helps in clearing a blocked nose. Have a stuffy nose? All you need to do is mix a little honey with steaming hot water in a basin and inhale the fumes that are coming from that basin, with a towel draped over your head. This will help clear your nose most effectively.

#45 It can be used to highlight your hair. Want to make your hair lighter? Leave it to the hydrogen peroxide that is found in honey. All you need to do is mix 3 spoons of honey with 2 spoons of water and apply it to damp hair. Then you need to let it sit for one hour before you wash it off.

Conclusion

We have seen over the course of this book, exactly how wonderful honey can be where it comes to providing a vast number of benefits that are really more than sufficient to help us make the right choice of replacing that sugar in our diet with the wonderful substitute that is honey. You will come to see that your health will improve substantially in the process and you will be extremely happy that you made the decision to covert to a honey-based diet.

We have always been told that foods that are found in nature are far healthier than those that are processed, so why not make this the moment to take this piece of advice a lot more seriously?

Yes, go to that trusted supermarket today itself and make sure that you get your first week's supply of honey – you'll be certainly glad you did! In time you will forget all about sugar, and wonder why on earth so many people out there are so dependent on it. If you really have to be dependent on something, then let it be honey!

Your Free Gift

I am really grateful and thankful for your purchase. As a small symbol of my appreciation, I would like to give you my FREE book on Essential Oils so you can begin to use them in your life.

In my essential oils: 100+ Essential Oils for beauty, healing, personal care, and detox ebook, you will find various ways and methods that will help you to use essential oils and get results RIGHT NOW. You will also get all my new ebooks at a discounted price ☺

Here is the link for the ebook:

Download Now